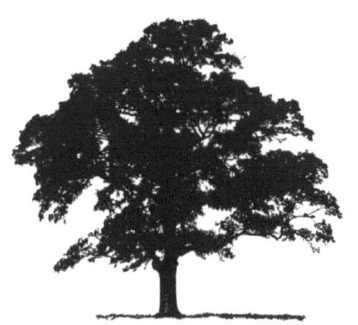

Siggie the Sloth's Sensory Adventures
Delicious Discoveries

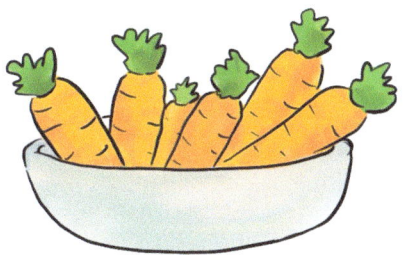

Natalie Morgan & Melanie laCour

Illustrated by Nita Candra

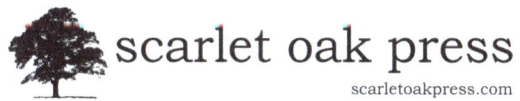

scarlet oak press

scarletoakpress.com

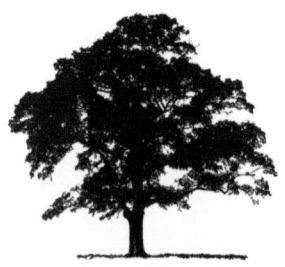

scarlet oak press.

For permissions and information about special discounts for bulk purchases, contact Scarlet Oak Press at contact@scarletoakpress.com.

ISBN: 978-1-954974-24-1 (eBook)

ISBN: 978-1-954974-27-2 (Paperback)

ISBN: 978-1-954974-23-4 (Hard Cover)

Library of Congress Control Number: 2025905255

Published by Scarlet Oak Press (scarletoakpress.com)

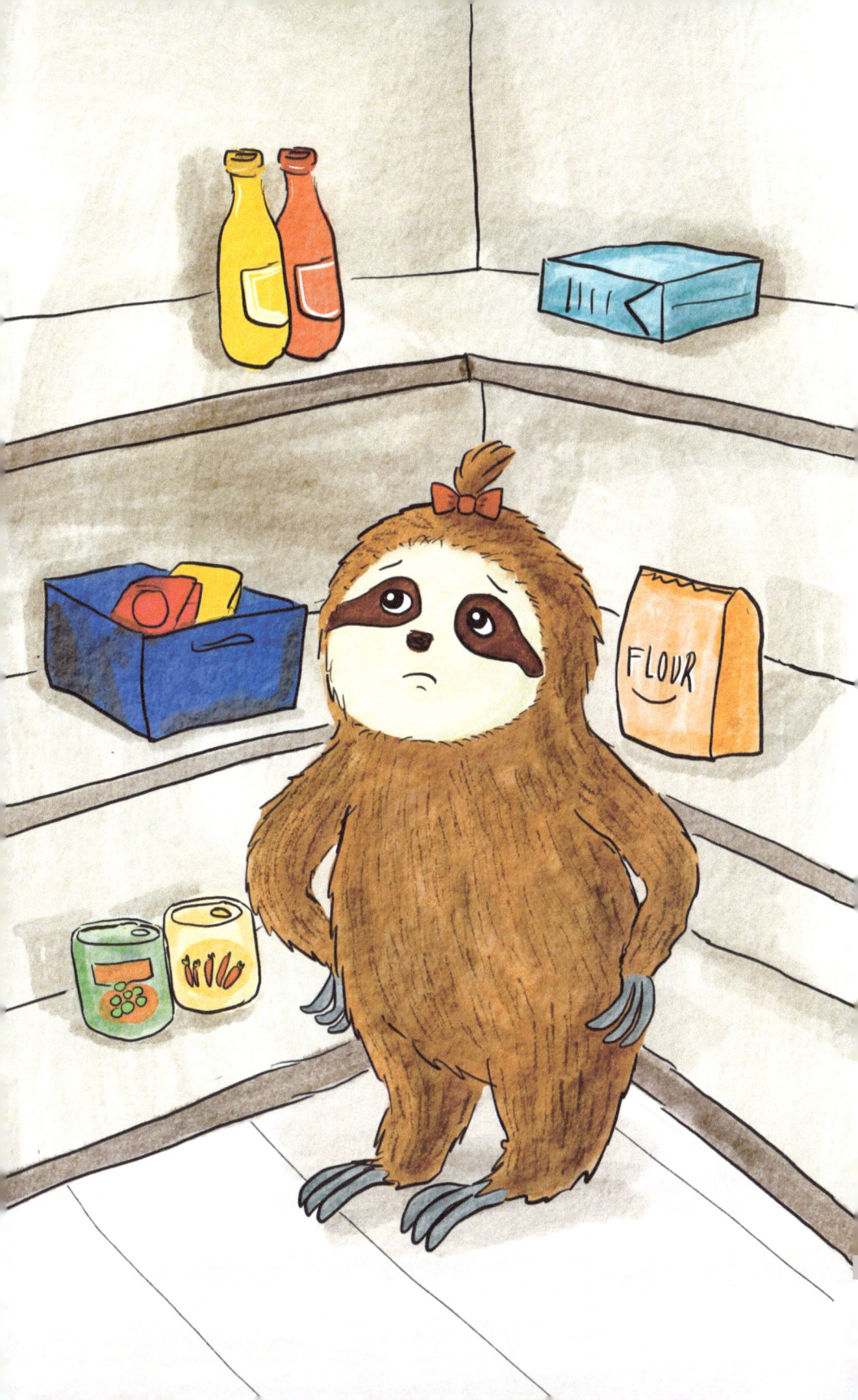

This book is dedicated to
Lily, Talia, Tripp, and August.

Siggie's tummy rumbled.
She was so hungry, but what could she eat?

She searched through the pantry
but didn't see any of her favorites.

No animal crackers.
No goldfish. No fruit snacks.

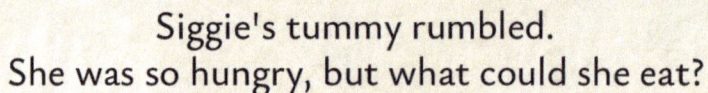

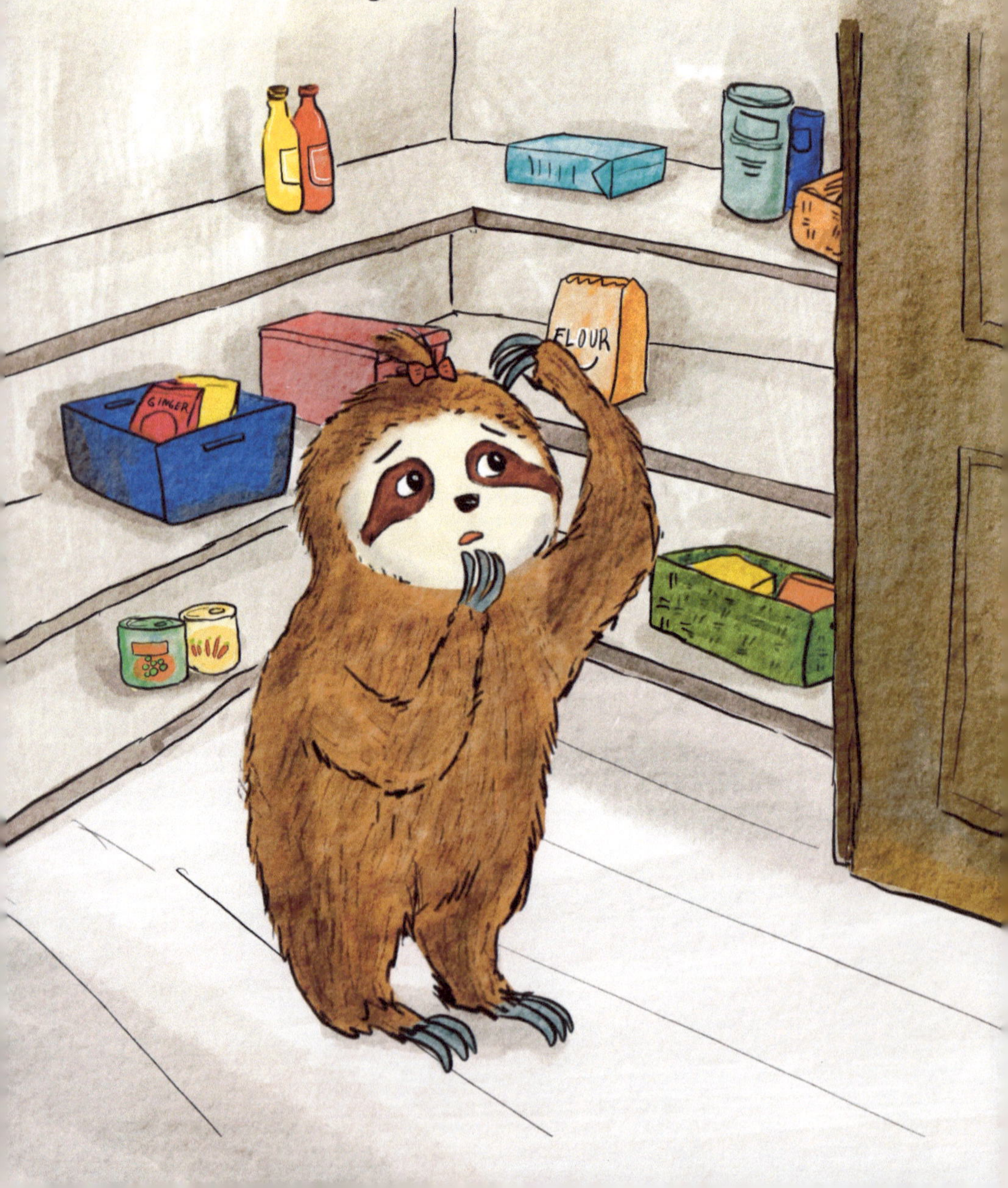

"This is hopeless!" sighed Siggie as she prepared to wither away.

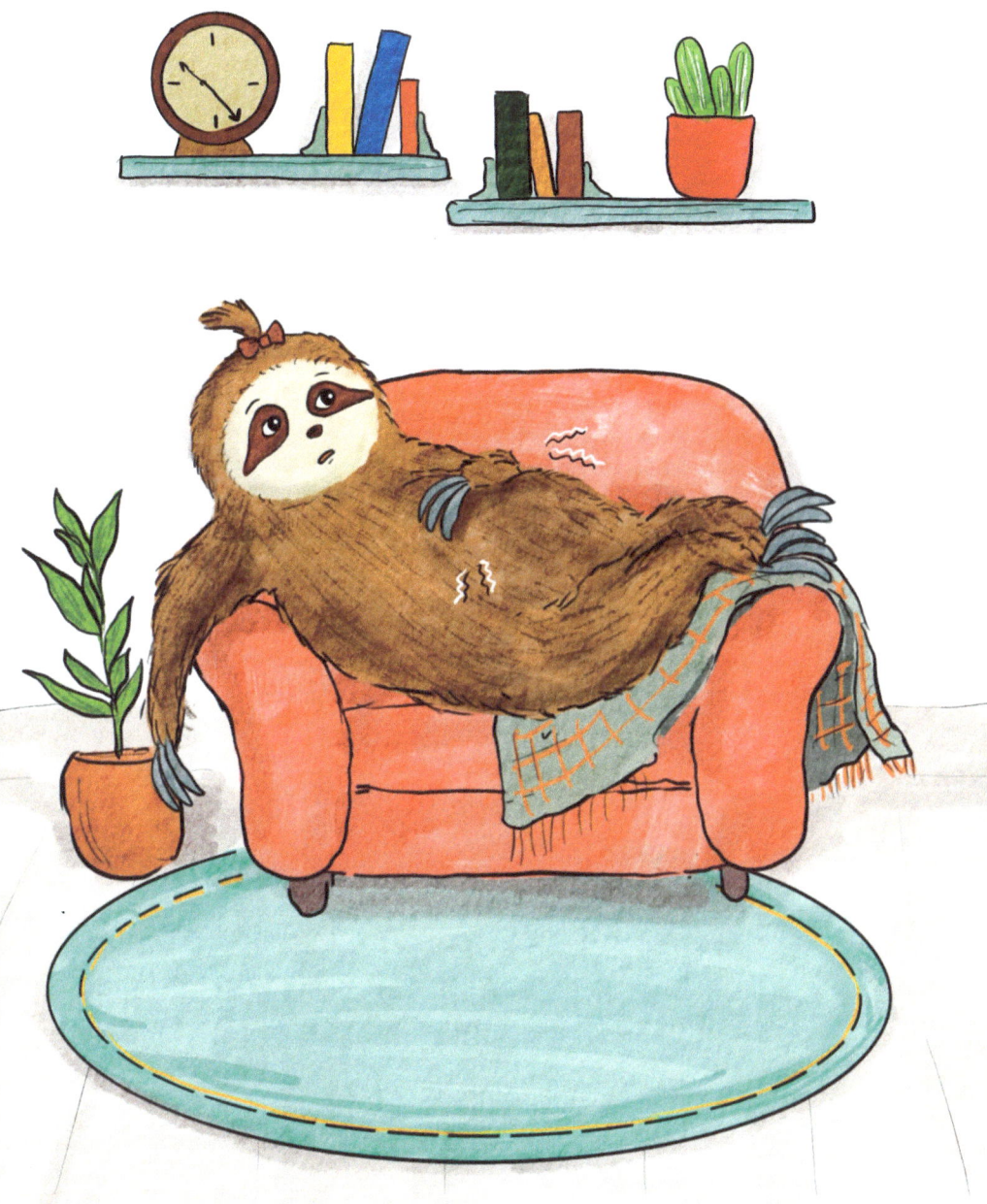

Then, as her tummy rumbled again, Siggie said, "This is silly. I can't go hungry in a kitchen full of food."

Siggie remembered how much she liked adventure. "I could have an adventure right here in the kitchen. A new food adventure!"

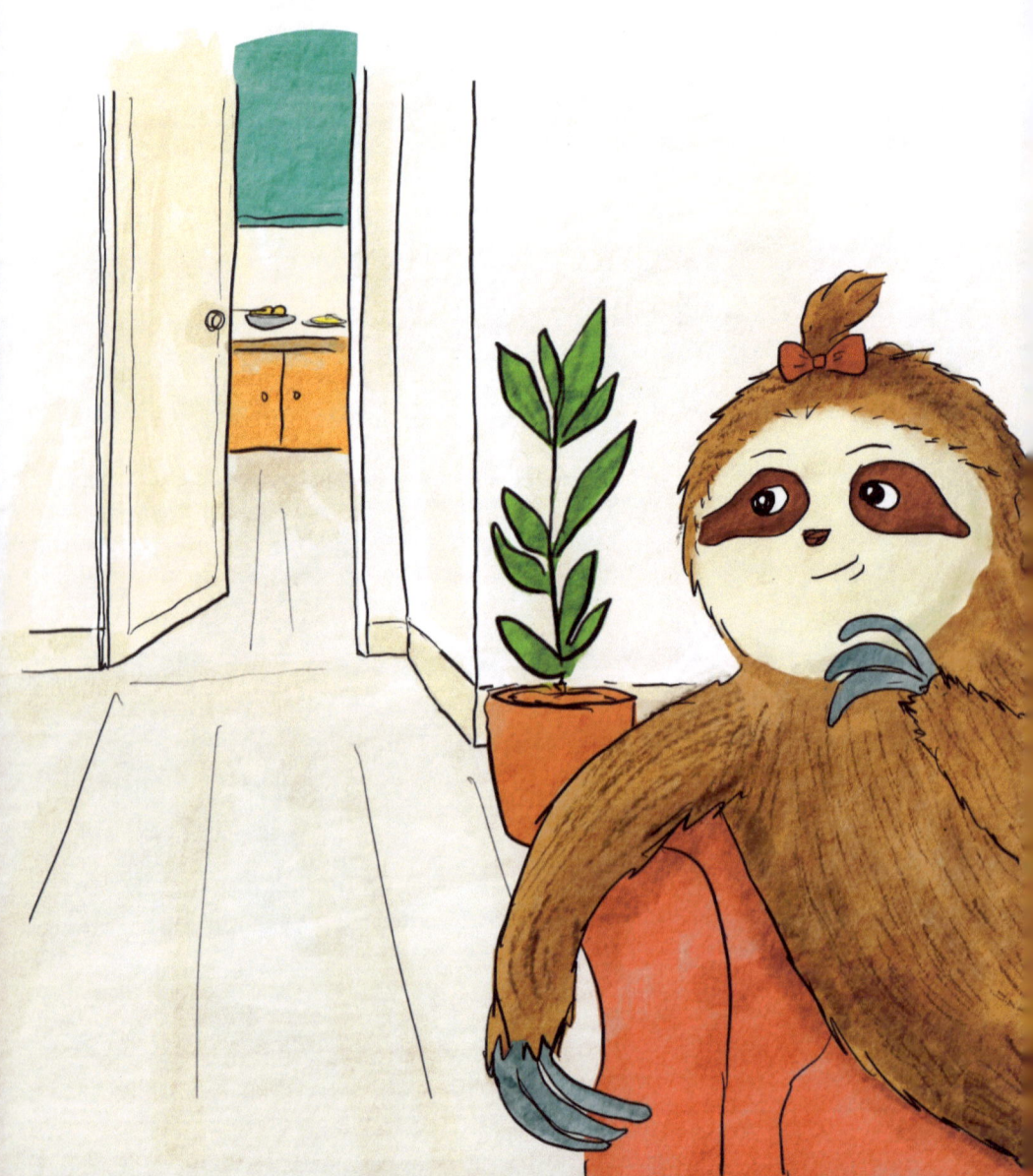

Today was the day she would have the courage
to try some unfamiliar foods--but how?

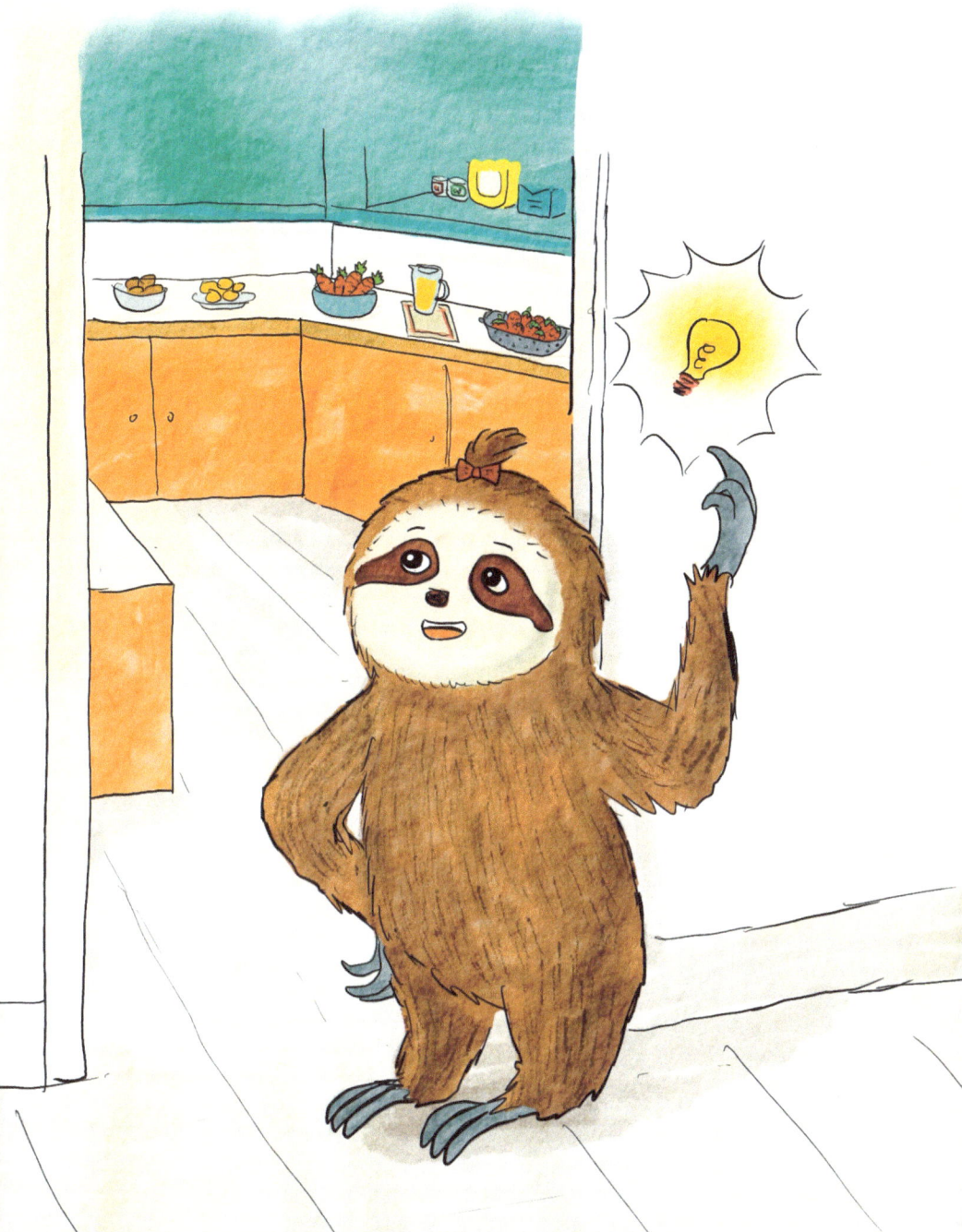

Her teacher had explained that people experience the world through the body's five senses: sight, sound, taste, smell, and touch.

Everyone's senses are unique, and not everybody has all five.

Siggie would experience her world through them!

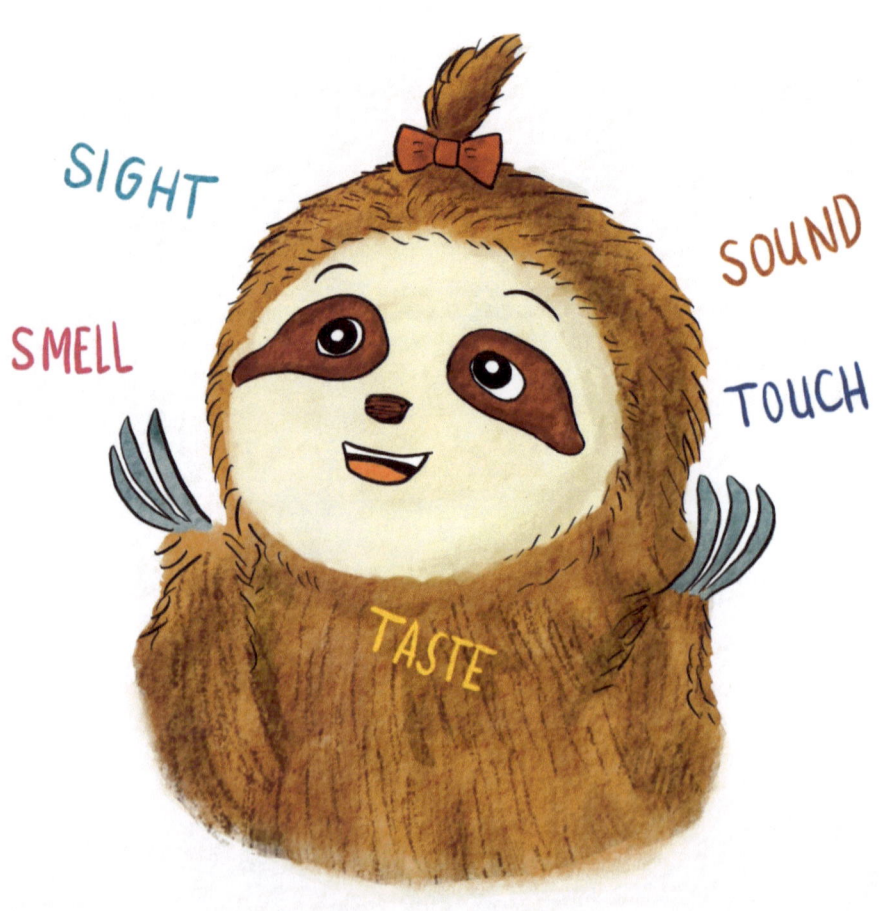

SIGHT

SOUND

SMELL

TOUCH

TASTE

So, Siggie prepared to be brave.

Strange shapes, smells or textures would not keep her from tasting a new taste.

She was ready to dig in!

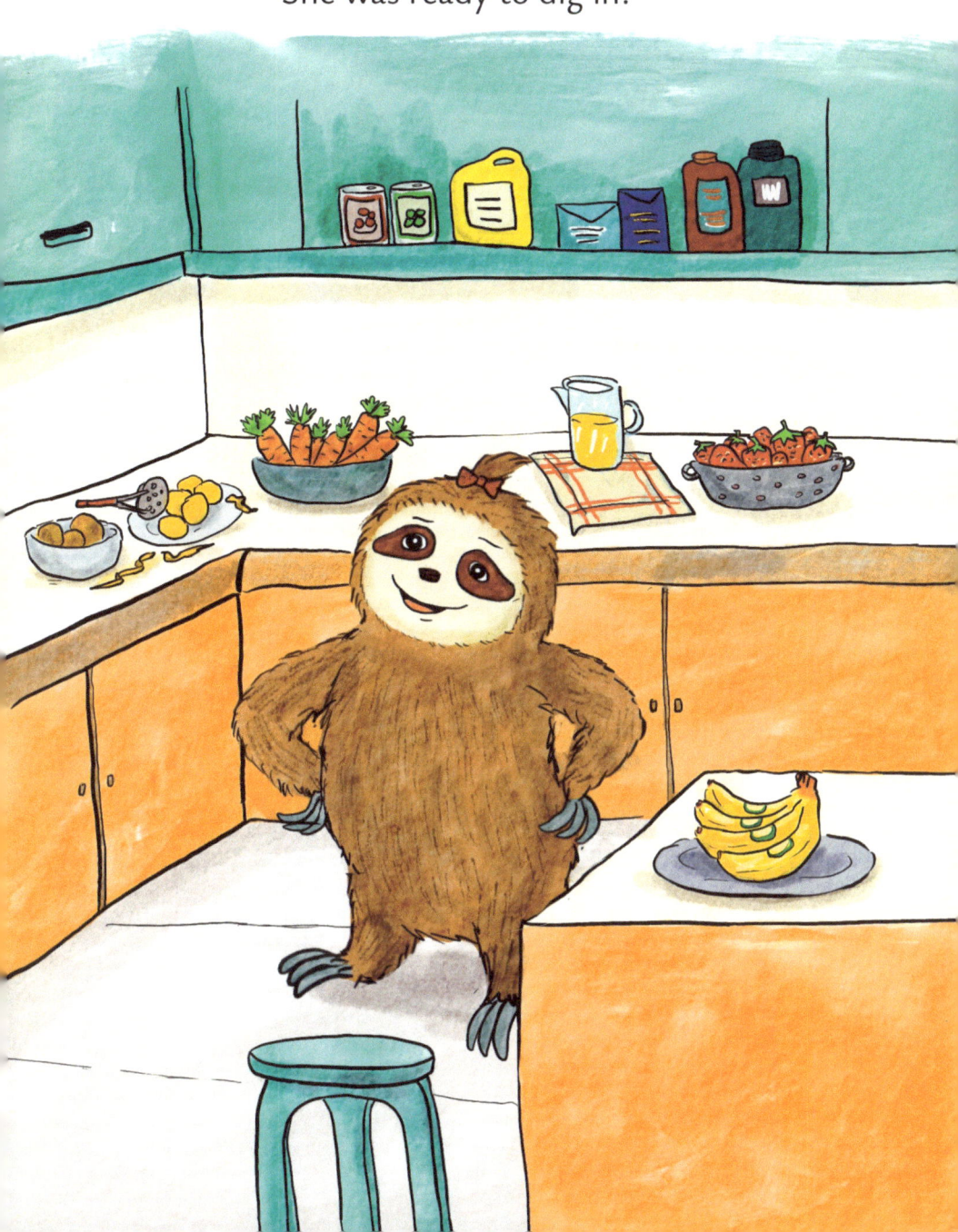

Siggie saw a pot full of fluff
asking out loud, "What is this stuff?"

She felt the misty, hot steam rise
brushing her cheeks and clouding her eyes.

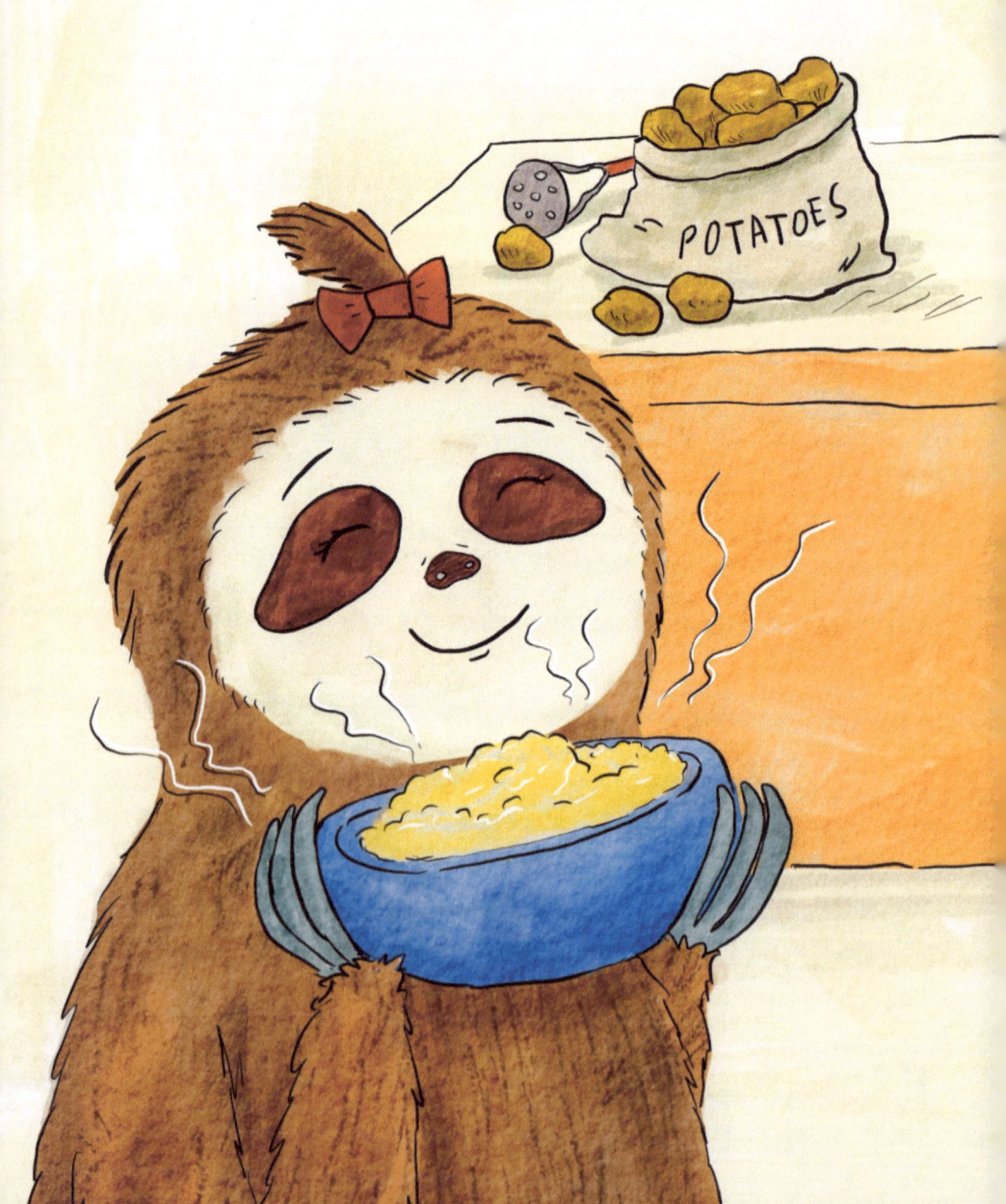

Siggie smelled the earthy air
as she sat down in her favorite chair.

She heard the sound of a squashy squish
digging her spoon into the dish.

Siggie tasted the dense and starchy puff
eating 'til she'd had enough.

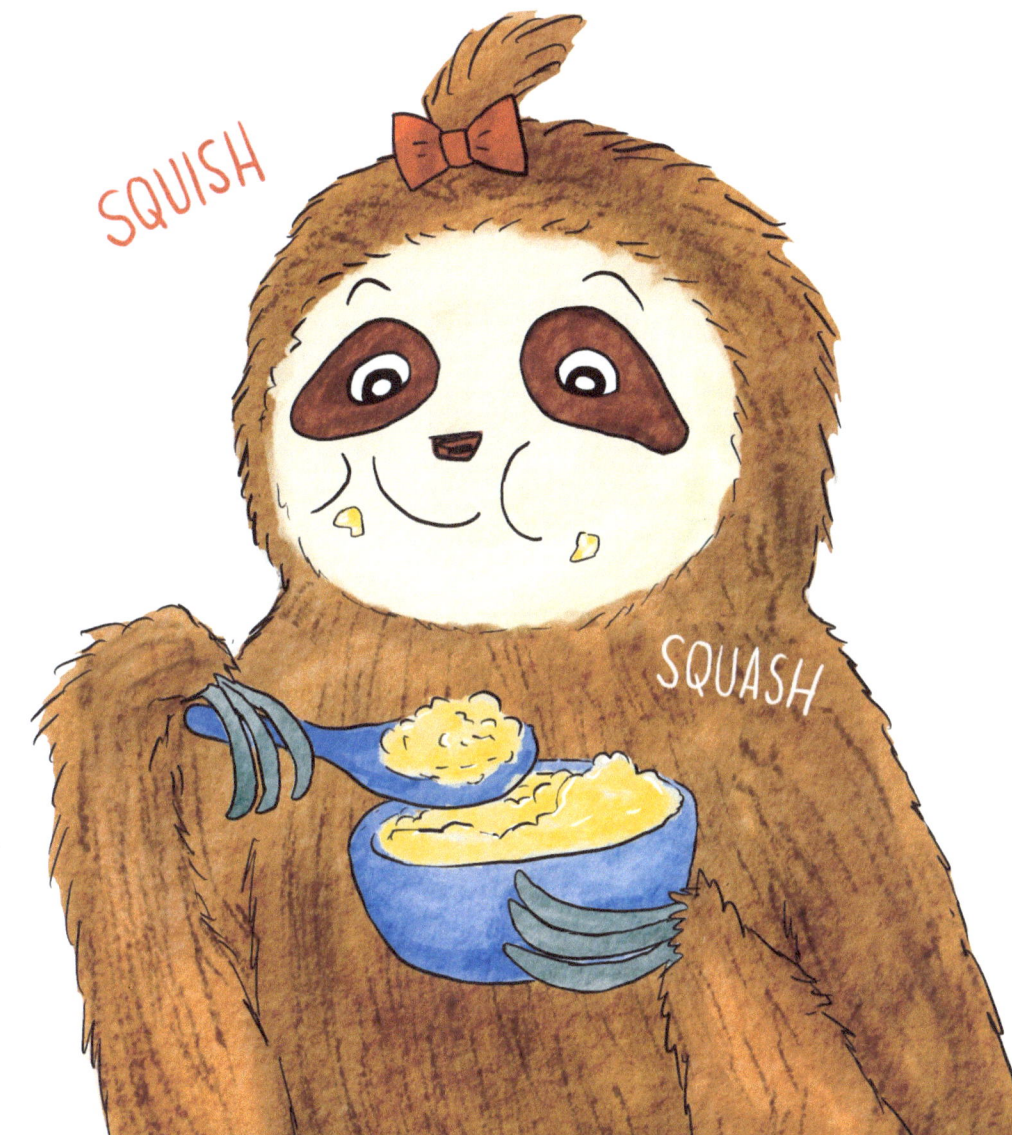

Siggie heard a munching crunch
when she went to feed her rabbit lunch.
She spied some shapes--long, orange and skinny
tapered and round. Some big, some mini.

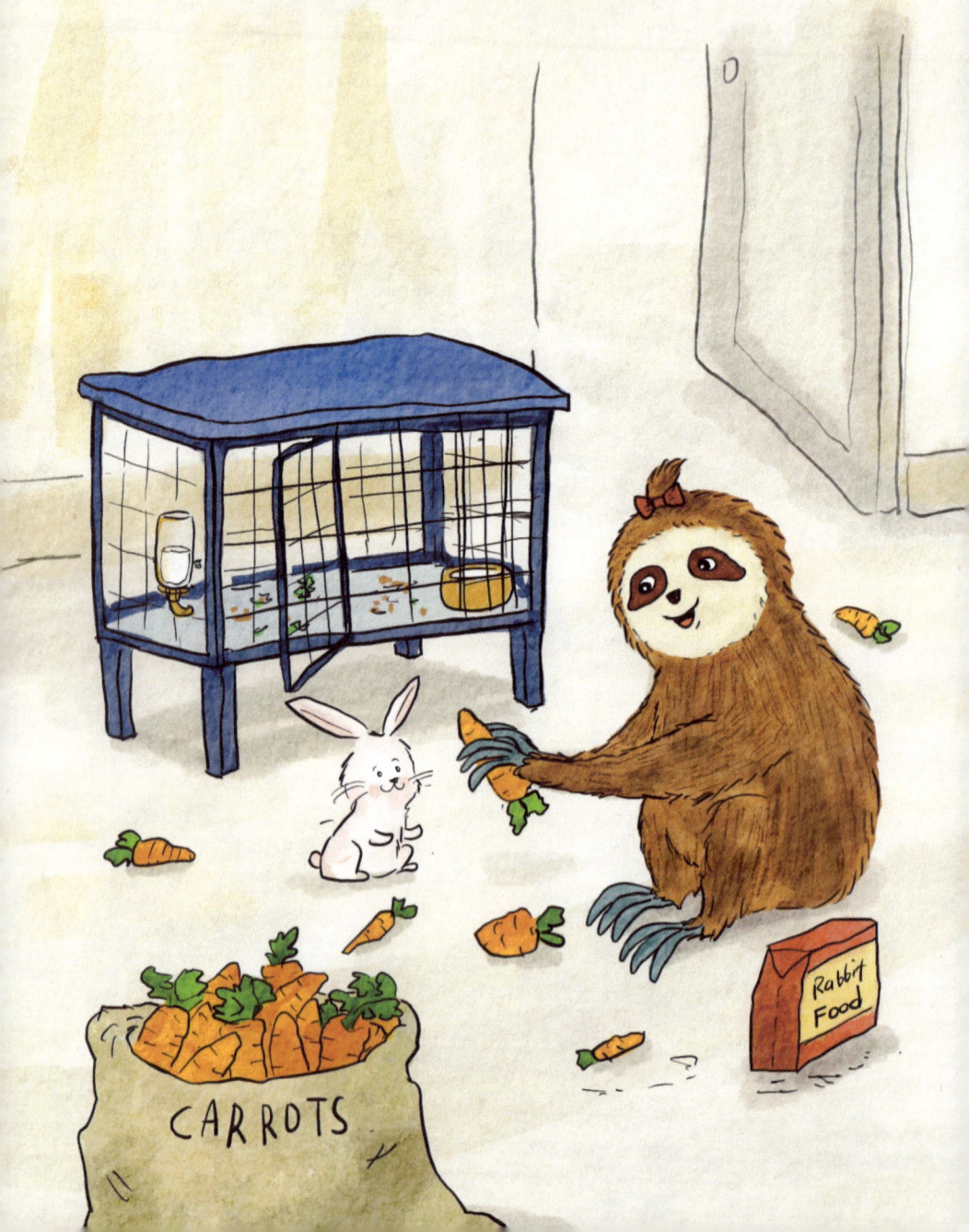

Siggie felt along the cool, smooth root
holding it sideways like a flute.

She inhaled the fresh and grassy smell.
Her rabbit's nose was twitching as well.

Siggie chomped down on a sweet, sharp bite.
For something healthy, these were alright.

SNIFF

Siggie craved something zingy to quickly devour
a tangy solid squish and flavor sweetly sour.

She scanned for the source of a zesty perfume
tracking the scent across the room.

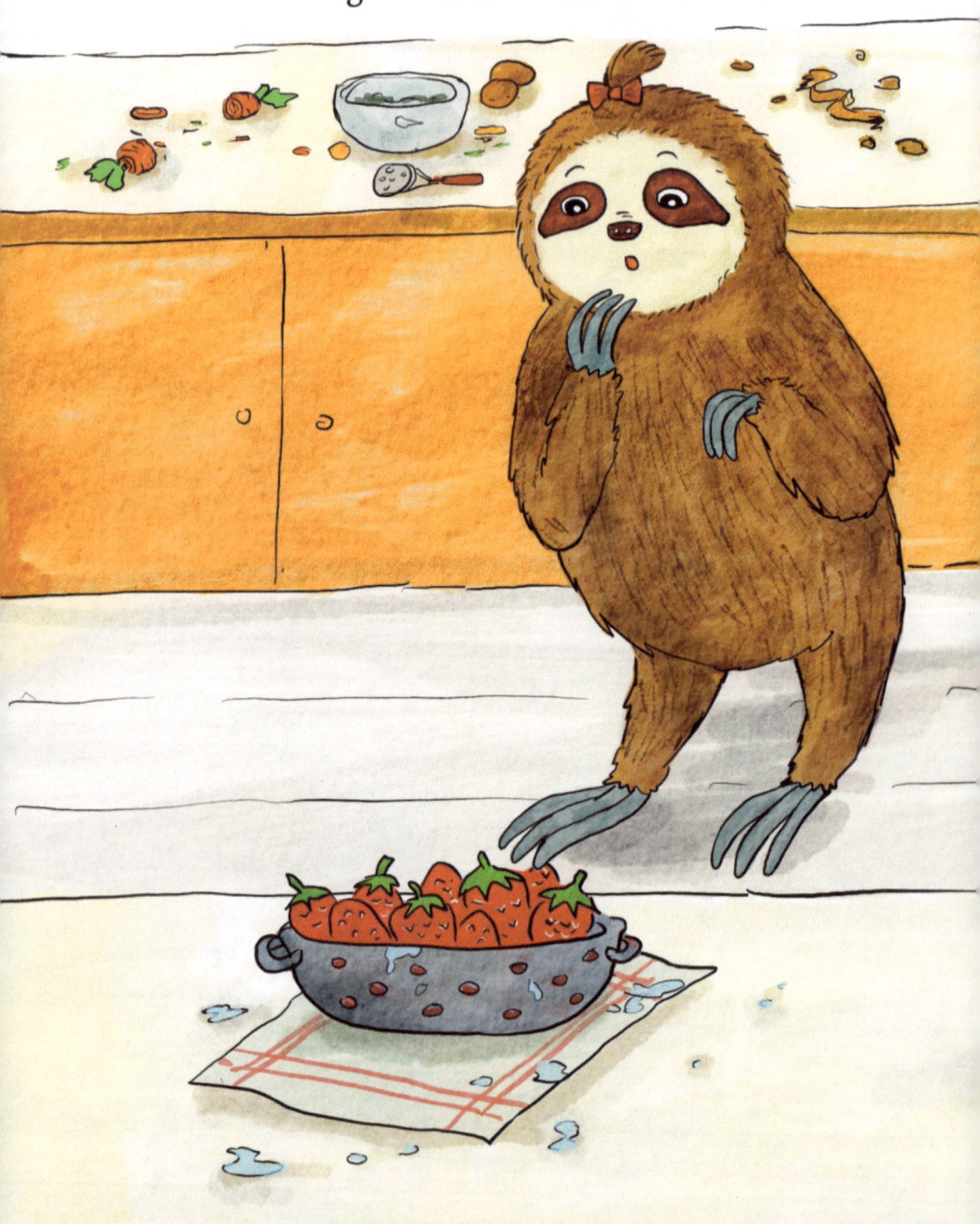

Siggie admired the sight of a red heaping pile
of heart-shaped flecked berries staining the tile.

She pinched one of the fruits by its green leafy crown
topping a coarseness she couldn't put down.

Siggie ground on the seeds with a grainy pop
tossing the cap aside with a plop.

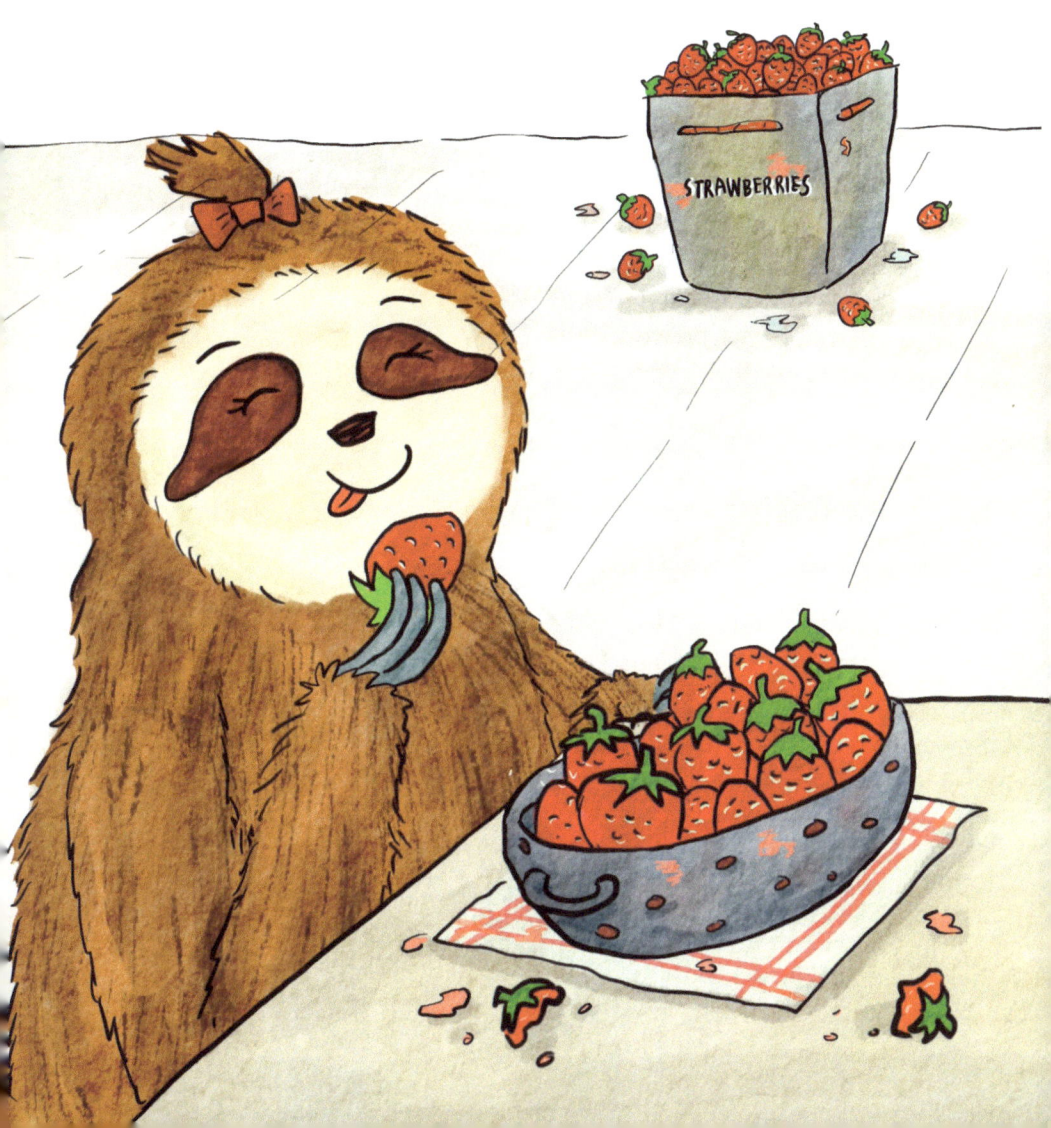

Siggie forked four small beads onto her tines
their green rounded shapes all straight in a line.

She enjoyed the gentle, beany smell
steamy and earthy from what she could tell.

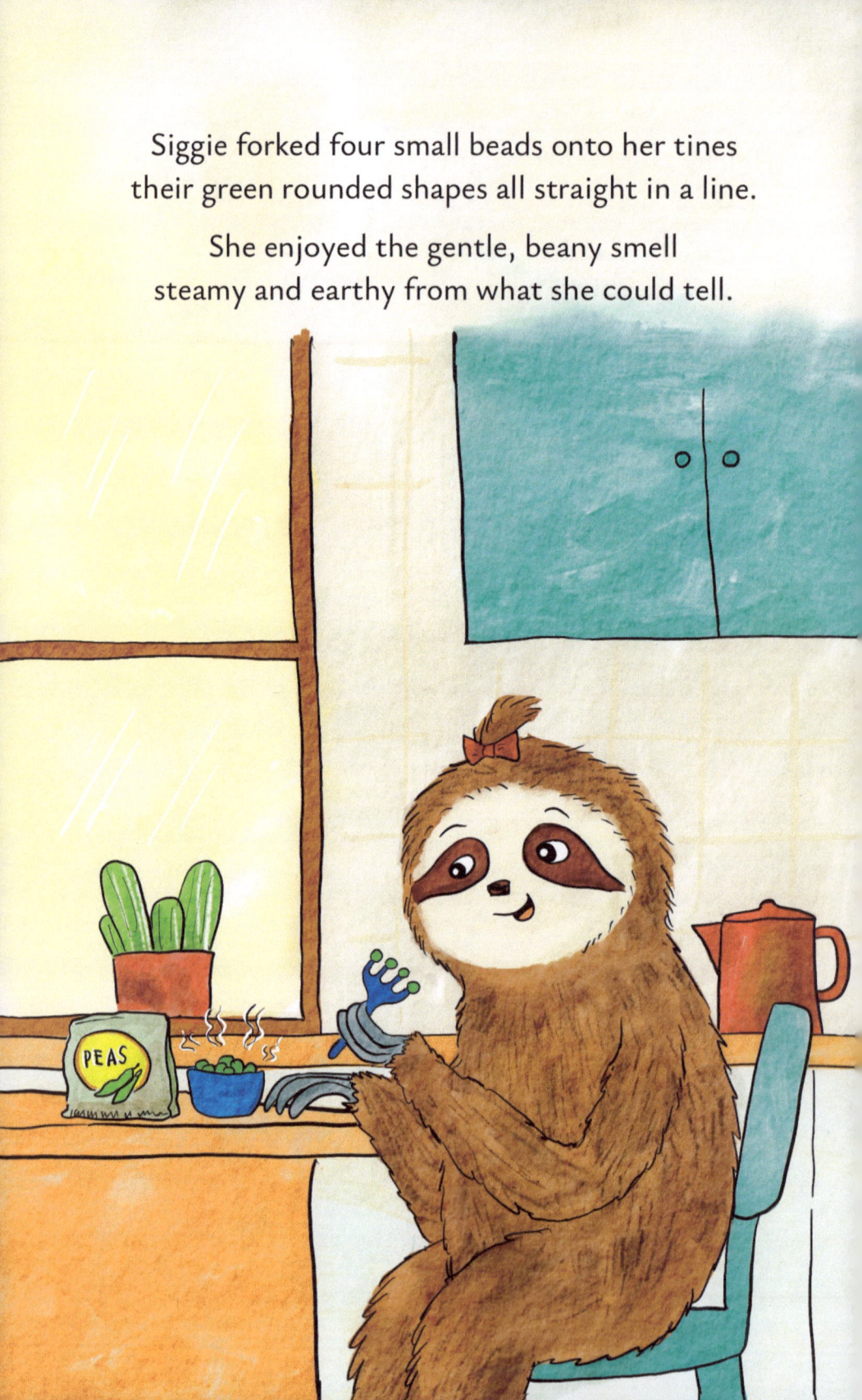

Siggie heard some quiet pip-popping bursts
crushed between her teeth at first.

She was proud of trying a new thing to eat
basic and ordinary, nutty and sweet.

Siggie chewed them into a pasty mush
smashing them down to a tacky smush.

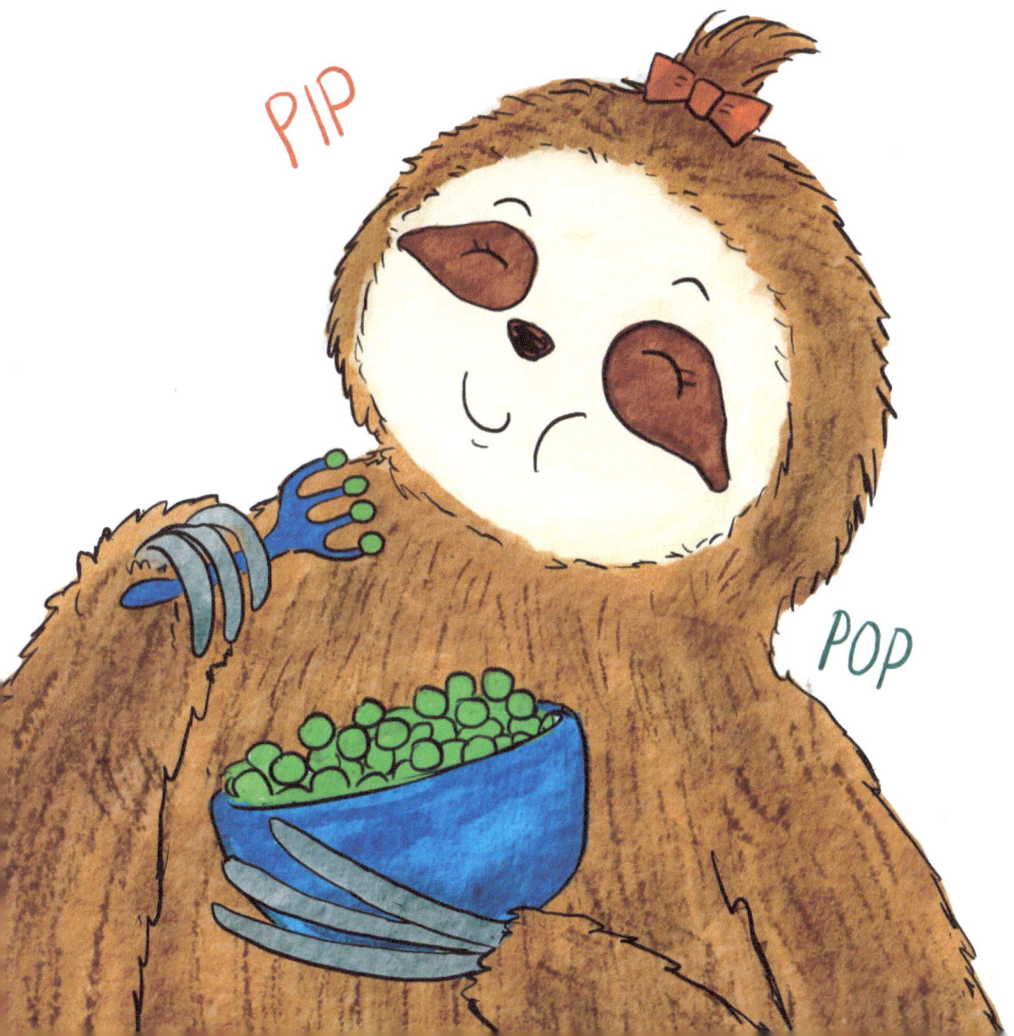

Siggie started to peel down the heavy smooth skin
to a solid gooey center hiding within.

She bit off a piece that was slimy and mellow
gumming it around like thick creamy Jell-O.

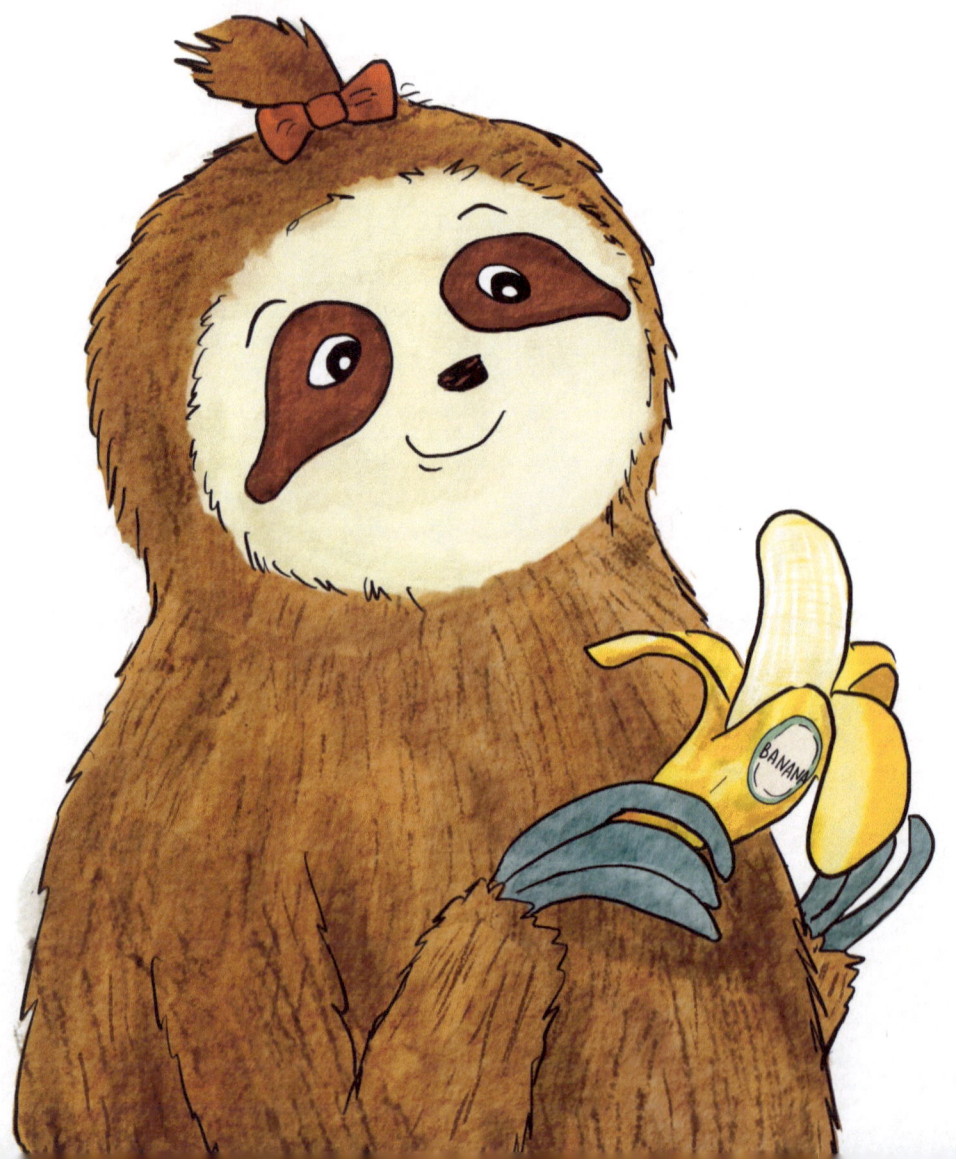

Siggie pondered the sound of this snack she adored
a sickly wet smacking that can't be ignored.

She liked that the outside was yellow and bright
a funny long shape that curved to the right.

Siggie noticed a smell that was fruity and strong
a neat pungent treat you can carry along.

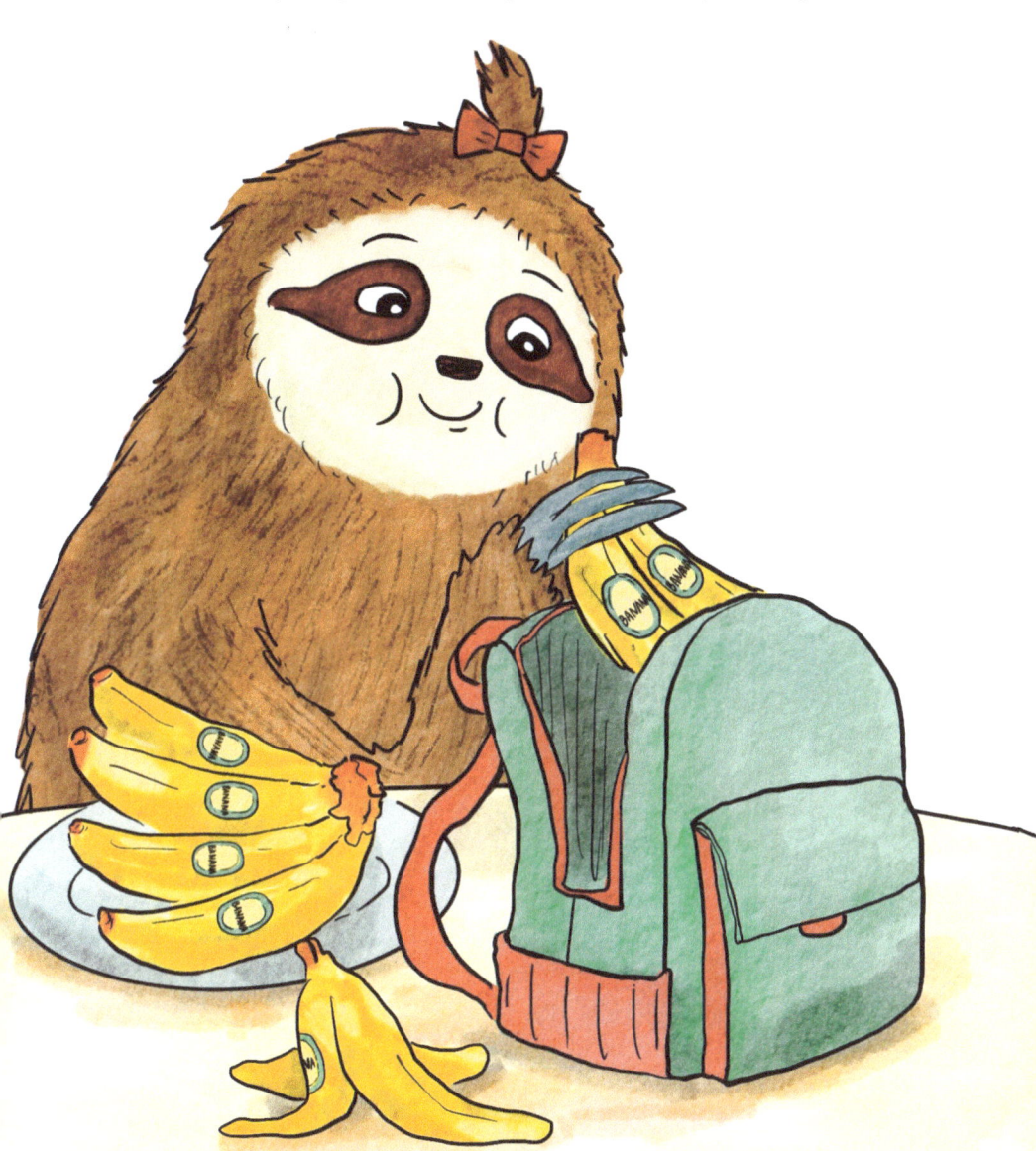

Siggie patted her full tummy.

"What a filling adventure!"
she thought as she let out a small burp.

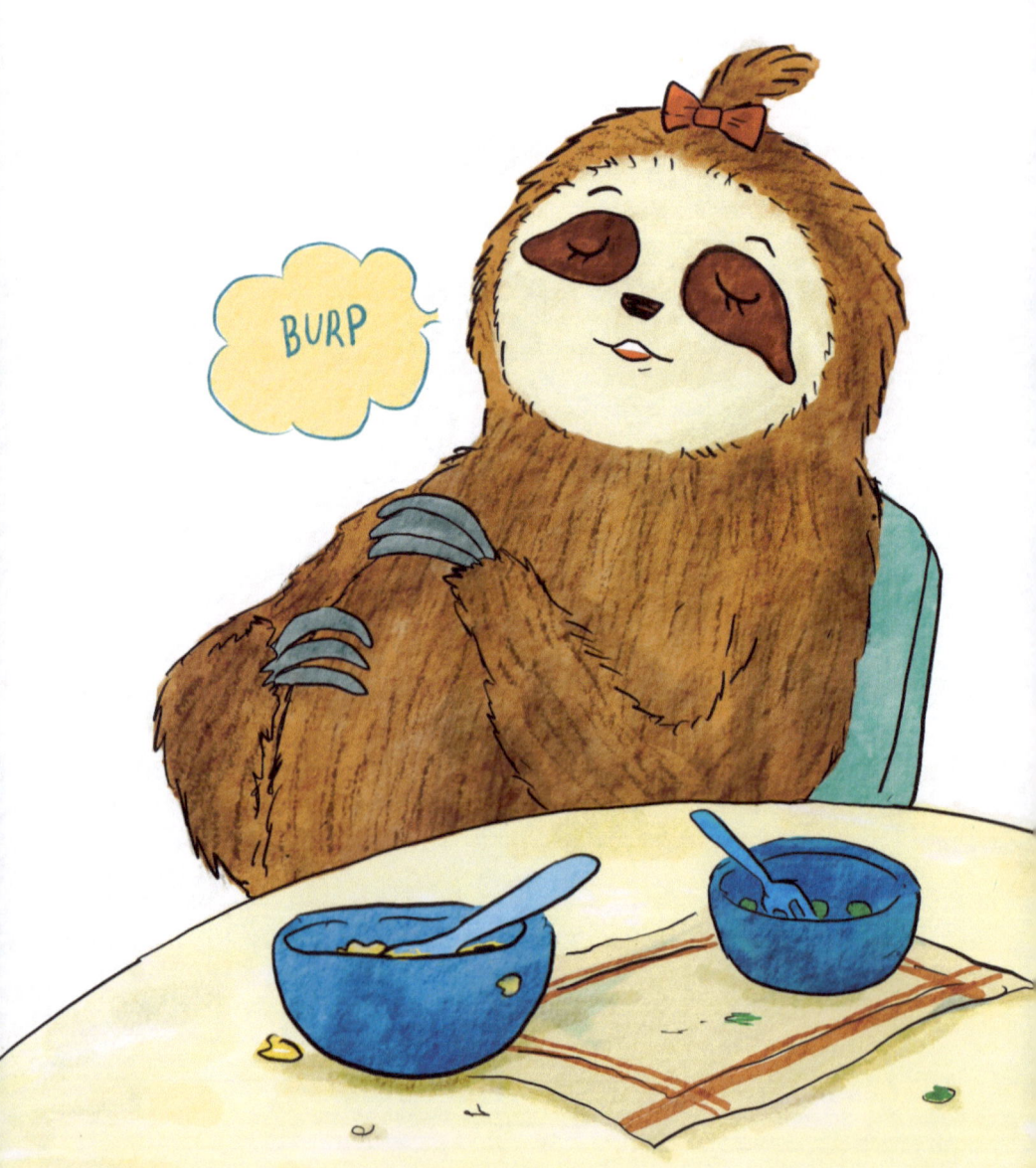

Now, Siggie was drowsy.

It takes a lot of energy to be brave and try new things.

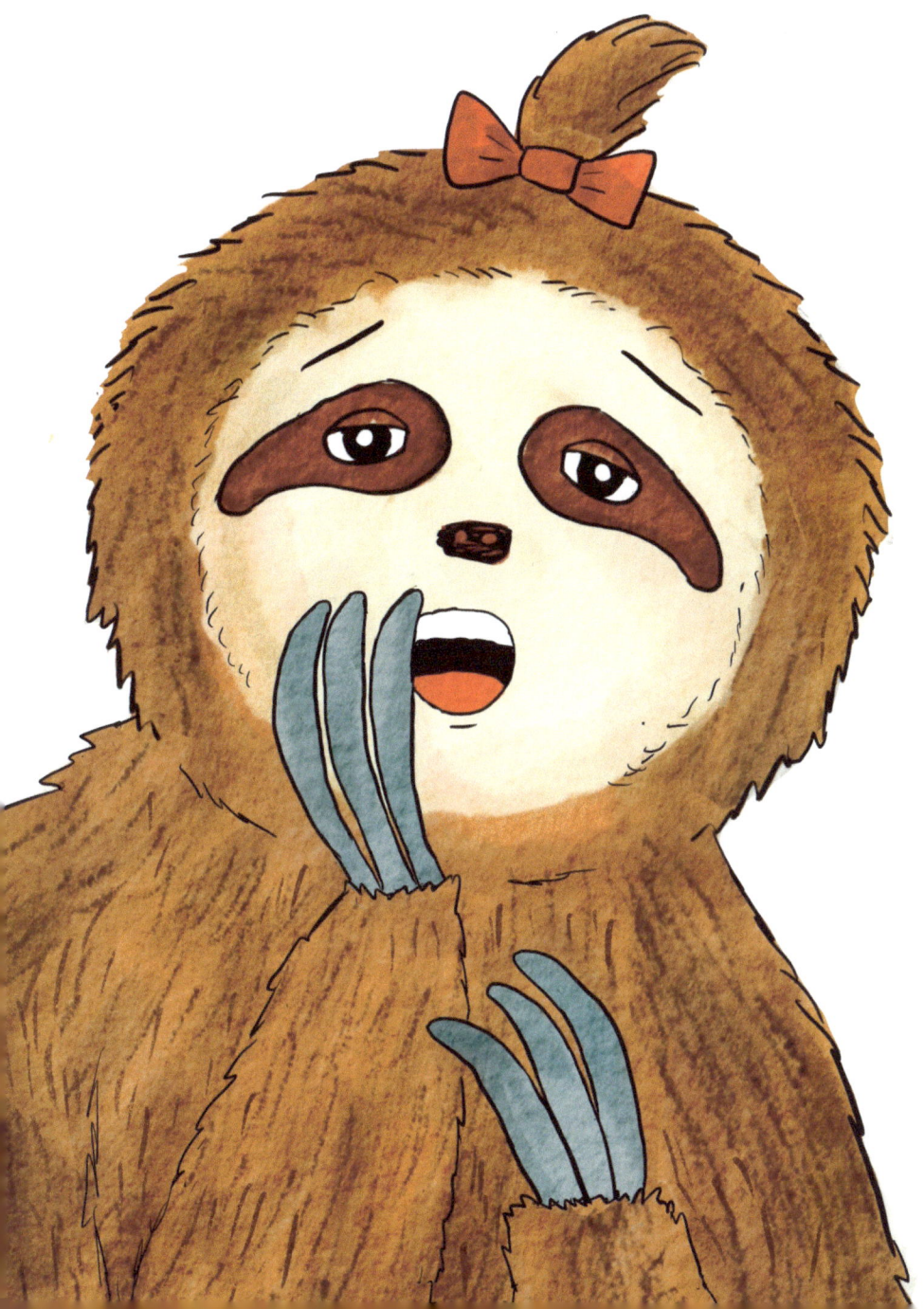

As Siggie lay in her comfy-cozy bed,
she thought about how proud she was of her courage.

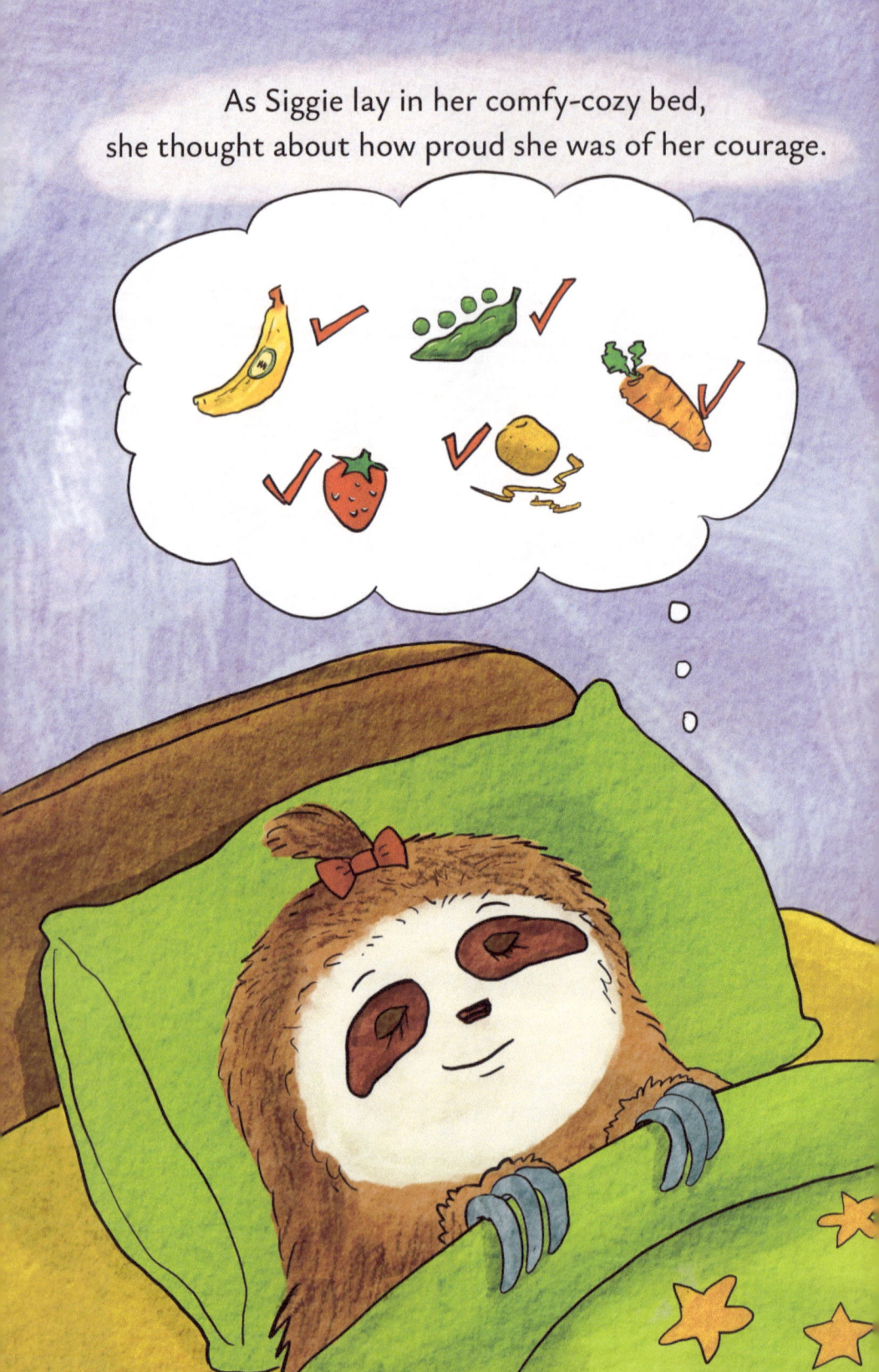

Tomorrow, Siggie would discover even more
new foods using all five senses.
Oatmeal, broccoli, cheese, scrambled eggs,
apples, and so much more!

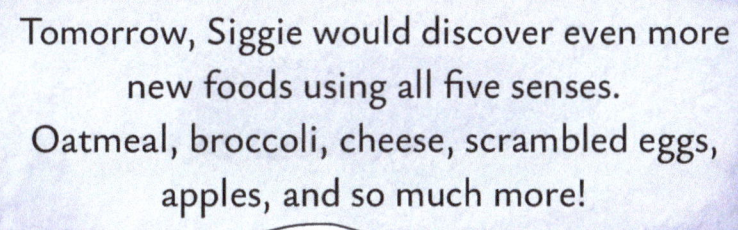

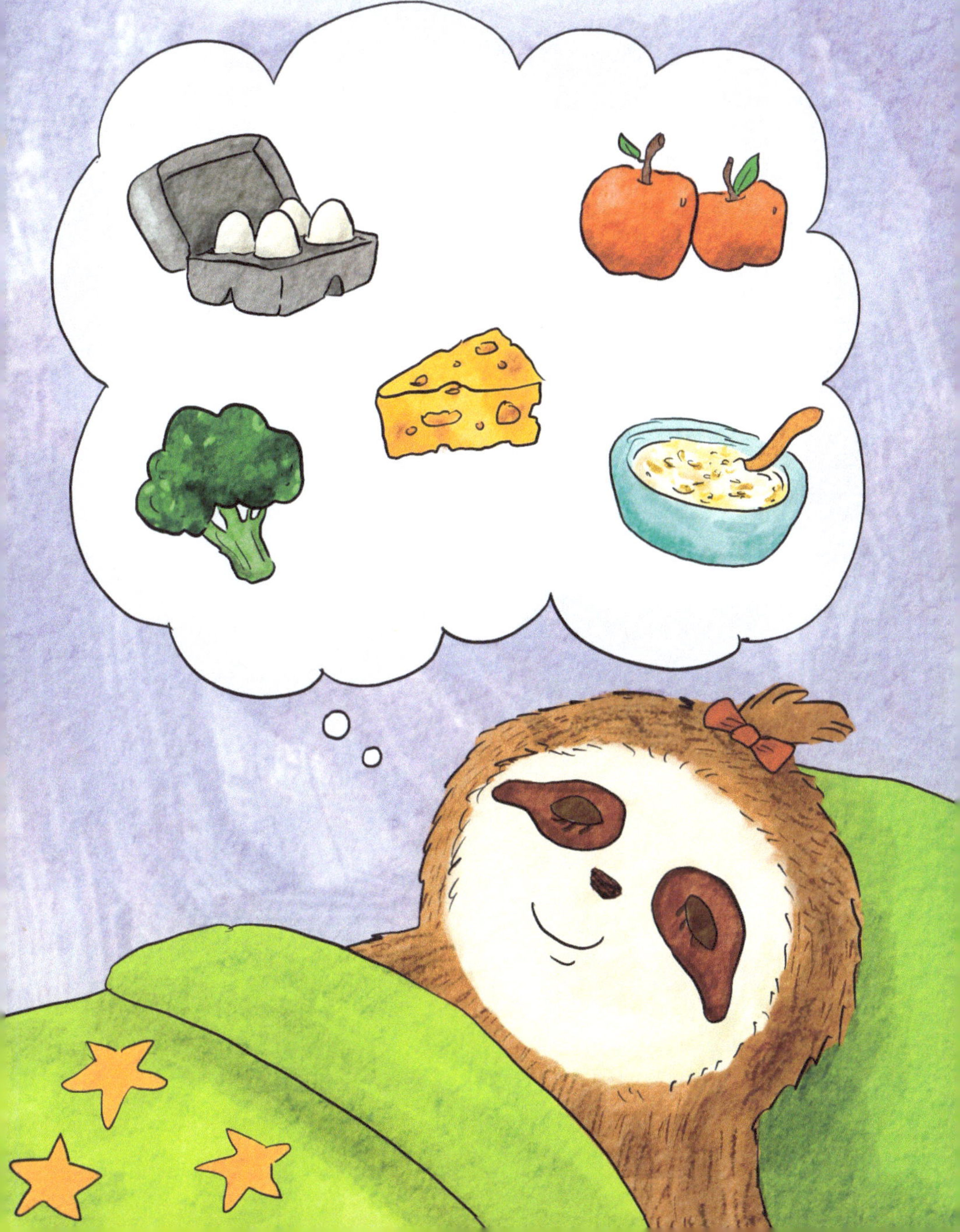

Her tummy rumbled just thinking about it.

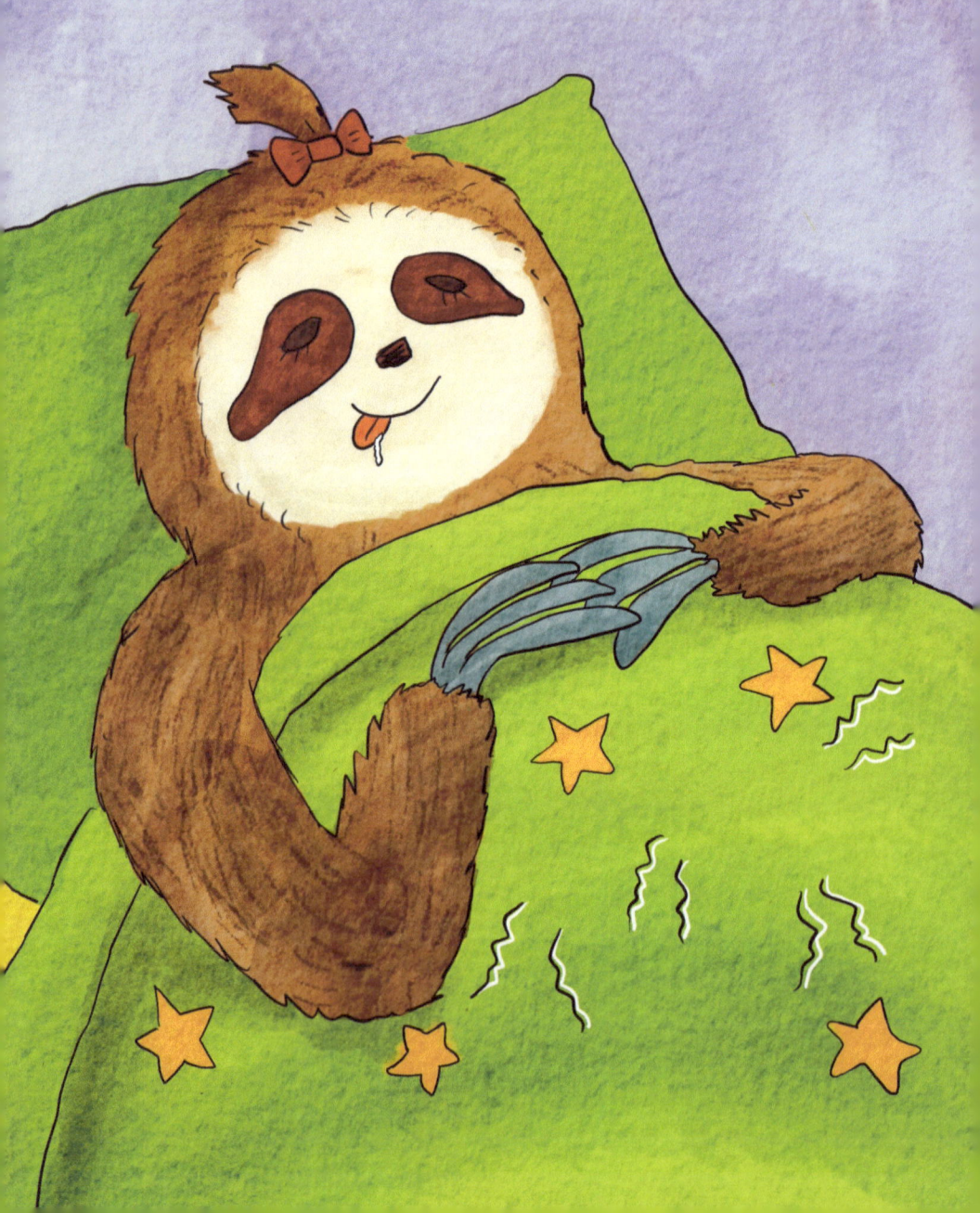

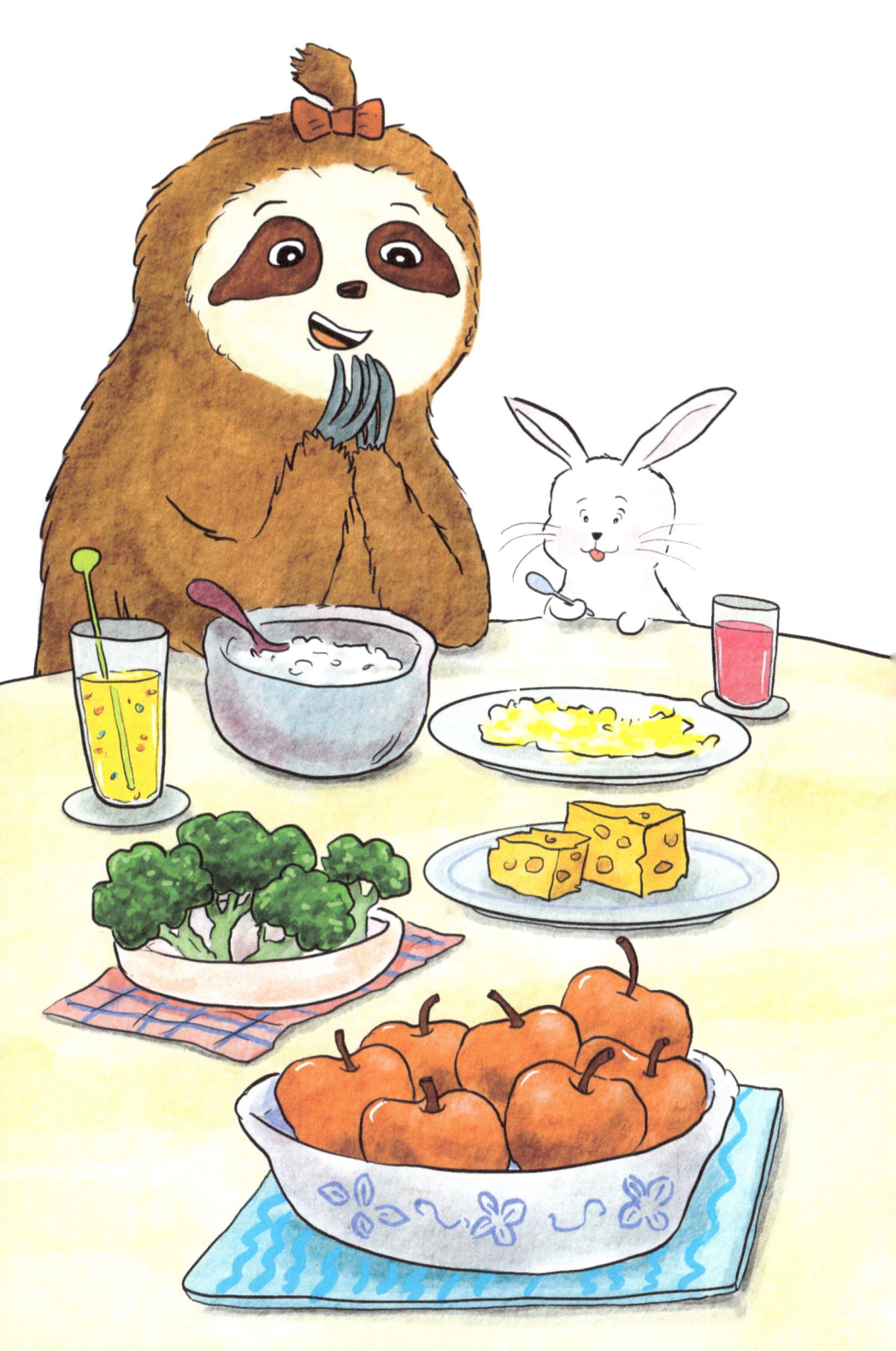

www.ingramcontent.com/pod-product-compliance
Lightning Source LLC
Chambersburg PA
CBHW040849120626
46547CB00001B/99